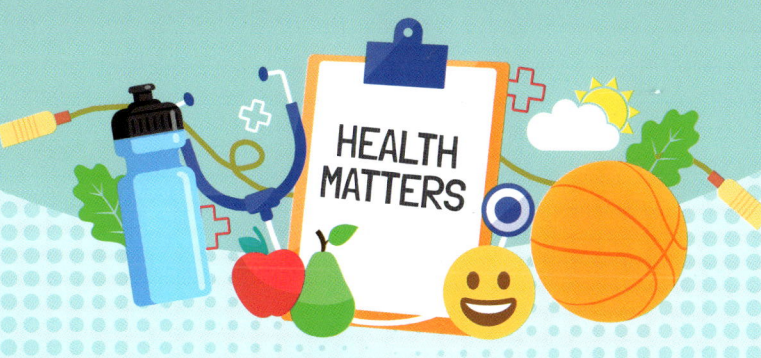

HEALTH MATTERS

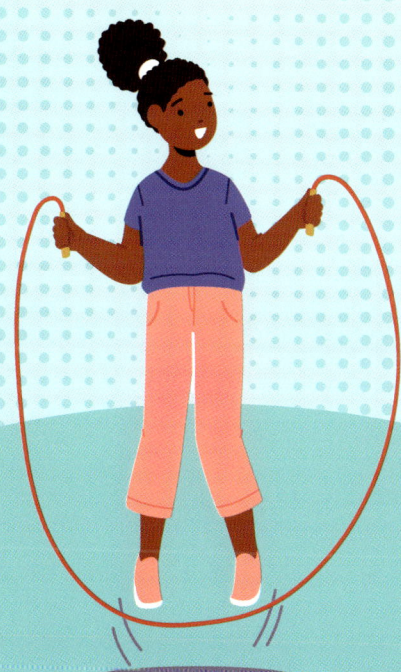

STAYING ACTIVE

Nancy Dickmann

Published by Brown Bear Books Ltd

4877 N. Circulo Bujia
Tucson, AZ 85718
USA

and

G14, Regent Studios
1 Thane Villas
London N7 7PH
UK

ISBN 978-1-83572-009-7 (ALB)
ISBN 978-1-83572-015-8 (paperback)
ISBN 978-1-83572-021-9 (ebook)

Library of Congress Cataloging-in-Publication Data available on request

Designer: Trudi Webb
Design Manager: Keith Davis
Children's Publisher: Anne O'Daly
Picture Manager: Sophie Mortimer

Picture Credits
Cover: Shutterstock: Good Studio, lemono and Shutterstock Vector Stock Library.
Interior: Shutterstock: Bahau 8, designisfine 4, GoodStudio 4, 5, 9, 11, 15t, 15r, Gvardgraph 12, Iconic Bestiary 20, lemono 1, 14, 17, Lioputra 16, Mus Illustrations 15br, PCH Vector 6, 21, Andrew Rylbalko 15bl, Jane Semina 18, StockSmartStudio 7, 15c, Tenstudio 7, 19, Vector_dream_team 10, Vector Juice 13, 15l.

t=top, b=bottom, l=left, r=right, c=center.

All other artwork, Brown Bear Books and Shutterstock Vector Stock Library.

Brown Bear Books has made every attempt to contact the copyright holder.
If you have any information about omissions, please contact: licensing@brownbearbooks.co.uk

Manufactured in the United States of America
CPSIA compliance information: Batch#AG/5662

Websites
The website addresses in this book were valid at the time of going to press. However, it is possible that contents or addresses may change following publication of this book. No responsibility for any such changes can be accepted by the author or the publisher. Readers should be supervised when they access the Internet.

Contents

Get Moving! 4

Why Be Active? 6

Staying Strong 8

How Much Is Enough? 10

What Can I Do? 12

Building Skills 14

Getting Ready 16

Power Up! 18

Active Together 20

Your Turn! 22

Find Out More 22

Glossary 23

Index 24

Get Moving!

Being active is a great way to keep your body healthy.

Your body can move in amazing ways. You can run and jump. You can wiggle and dance. Maybe you can even stand on your head! Being active means moving and using your body. It's a good way to stay fit and healthy.

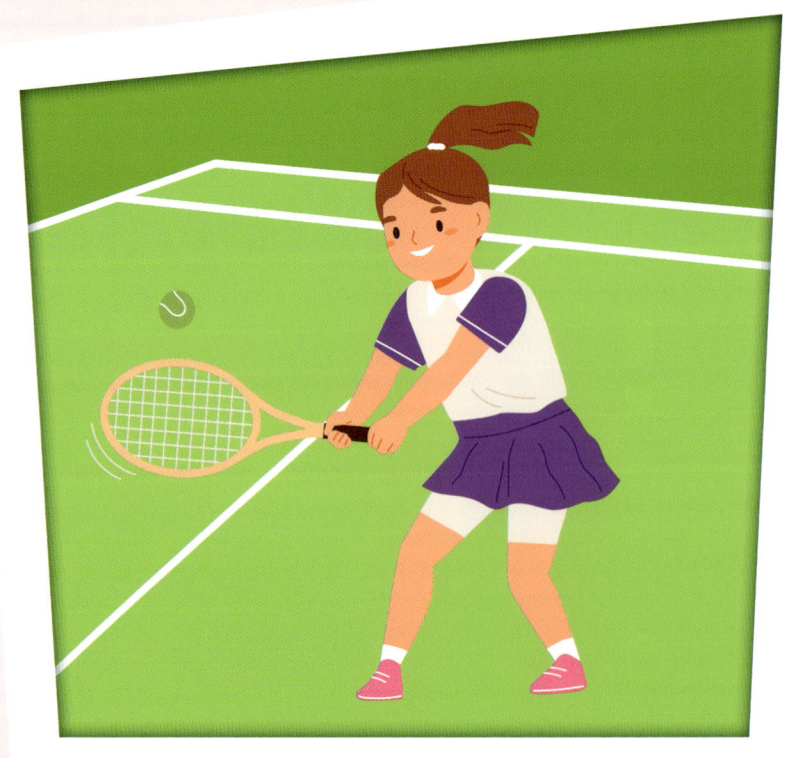

There are lots of ways to move your body.

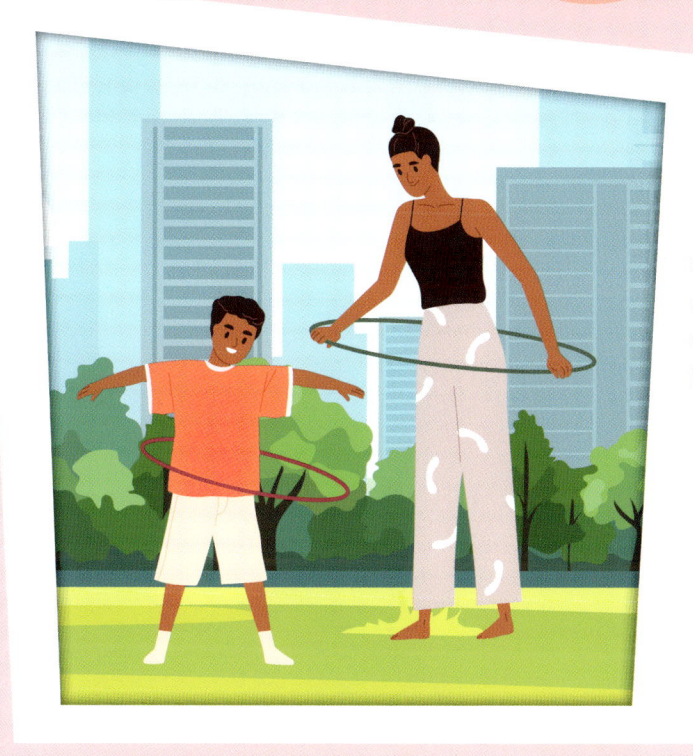

Staying active shouldn't feel like a chore. It can be a lot of fun!

In the United States only about **1 in 4 children** does enough physical activity every day.

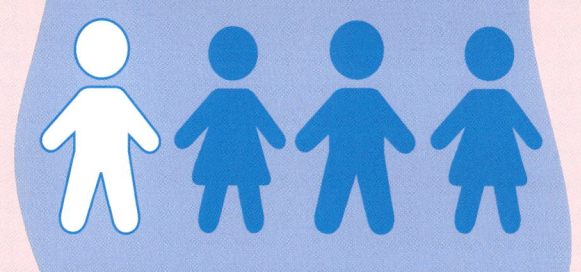

Everyday Activity

You don't have to run or play sports to stay active. Do you walk or bike to school? That counts. Dance party with your friends? That counts too! Even walking upstairs or doing some vacuuming gets your body moving.

Why Be Active?

Being active is good for your body. But how does it help?

A bicycle is really useful. But it won't work if the tires are flat or the chain is rusty. It has to be in good condition to work its best. And your body is the same! Keeping active helps your body work better.

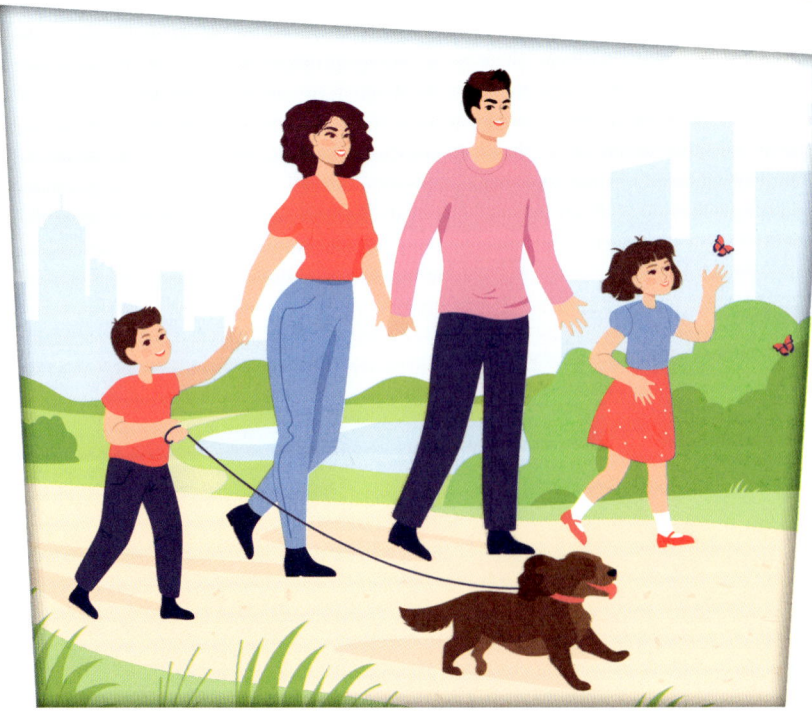

It's not just humans that need to stay active. Animals need exercise too!

Heart and Lungs

Your heart pumps blood around your body. Your lungs take in oxygen from the air. Then they pass it on through the blood. Exercise makes your heart and lungs work harder. This makes them stronger. They can do their jobs better.

Pump It Up

When you exercise, your muscles need more oxygen. Your heart beats faster. It pumps more oxygen-rich blood to your muscles.

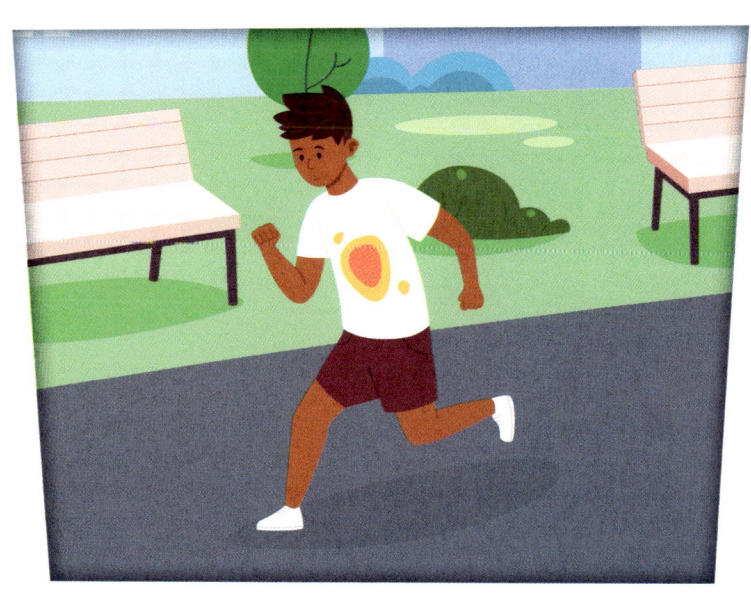

When you exercise, you breathe harder. This pulls more oxygen into your lungs.

Staying Strong

Exercise helps keep bones and muscles strong.

Your bones are tough and hard. They hold your body up. But bones can't move by themselves. That's what muscles do. They pull on bones to make your body move. Exercise helps your bones and muscles. The more you do, the stronger they get.

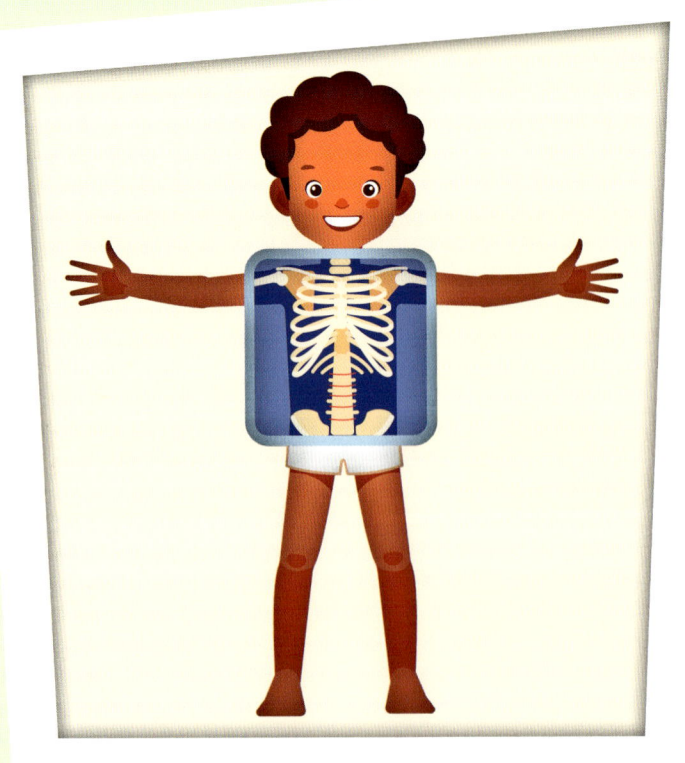

Your bones are inside your body.
They make a frame that holds you up.

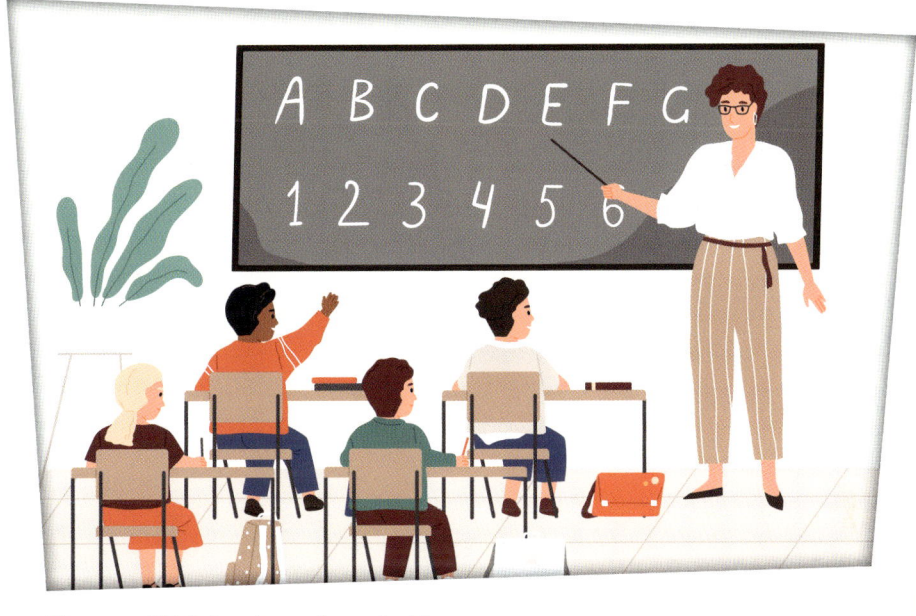
When you think hard, you learn better.
Exercise can help keep you focused!

Brain Boost

When you exercise, your body makes chemicals. They make you feel happy and relaxed. Exercise sends more blood to your brain. It helps you think better. But the effects wear off. That's why you exercise every day!

Which of these body parts does exercise help?

A. heart

B. brain

C. muscles

D. lungs

E. all of the above

How Much Is Enough?

Being active is really important. But how much exercise do you need?

Doctors say that you should do about an hour a day. Some exercise can be gentle, like walking. But some should be more energetic. Try to get your heart beating a bit faster. Panting or sweating show that your body is working hard!

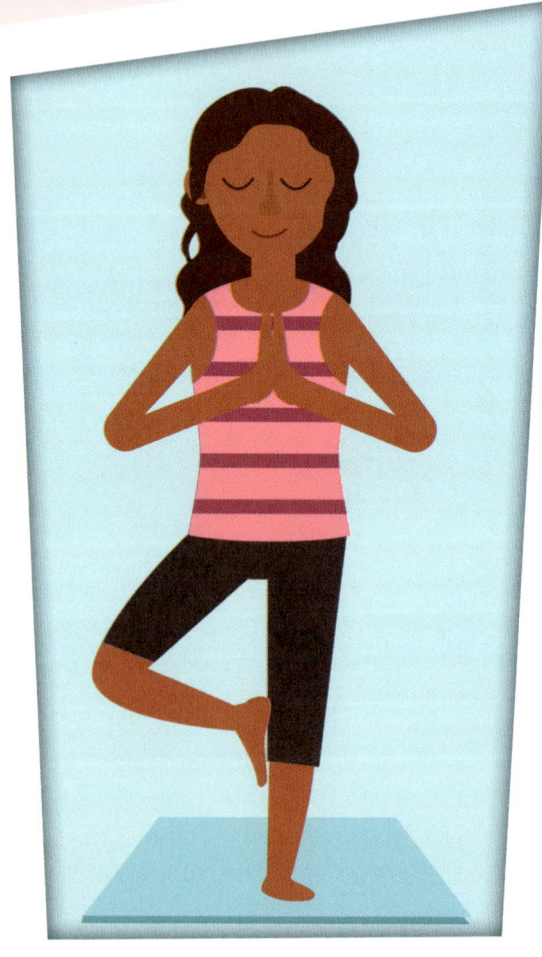

Yoga and gymnastics are great for keeping bones and muscles strong.

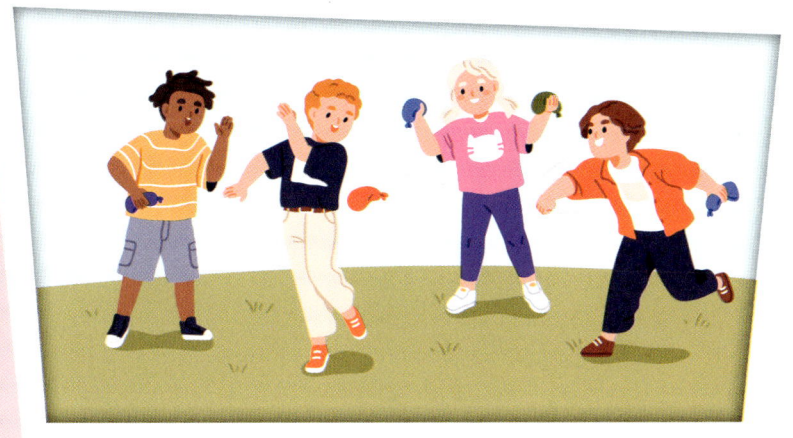

The more fun it is to be active, the more you'll do!

Adding Up

An hour a day might seem like a lot. But different activities all count! Did you ride a scooter to school? Did you play tag with your friends at recess? What about raking leaves with your dad, or walking the dog? It all adds up.

You can spread your activity throughout the day. How about:

* **20 minutes** walking
* **20 minutes** dancing at home
* **20 minutes** playing soccer at recess

What Can I Do?

There are lots of ways to be active.
Which one is your favorite?

Swimming is a great way to exercise. Running and fast walking are also good for your body. If wheels are your thing, ride a bike or scooter. You could even hit the skate park! Dancing, climbing, playing, and gym class count too.

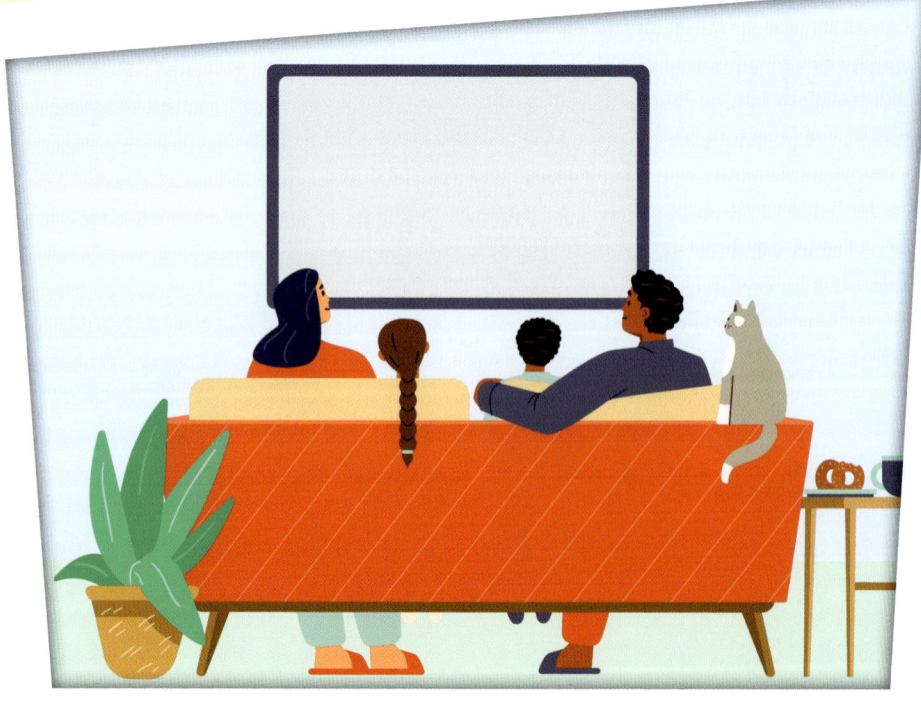

Put TV commercial breaks to good use. How about a jumping jacks contest?

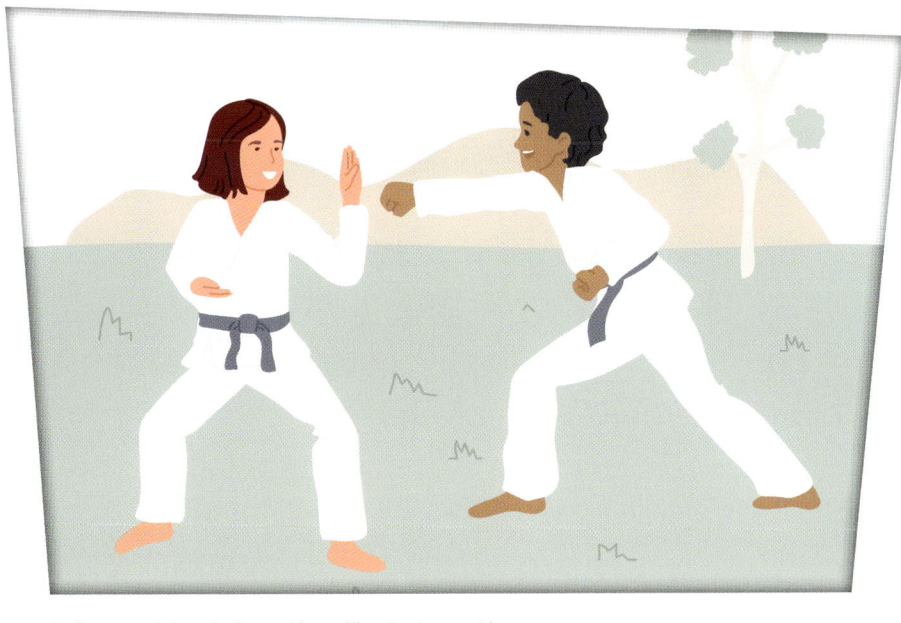

Ask your friends how they like to be active.
Maybe you could learn a new skill with them.

Twice as Nice

You don't have to be active on your own. Doing it with friends is even more fun! See if your friends want to play soccer or baseball. If it's a smaller group, play basketball or hit a tennis ball around. How about jump rope or playing catch?

Mix It Up!

Some activities make you breathe hard. They are good for your heart and lungs. Others are about strength and flexibility. They are good for muscles and bones. Try to get a mix of both types.

Building Skills

Exercise keeps your body healthy.
It also helps improve your skills!

Can you touch your toes? How good are you at balancing on one leg? Can you throw a ball and hit a target? How high can you jump? These are all physical skills. Exercise can help you get even better at them.

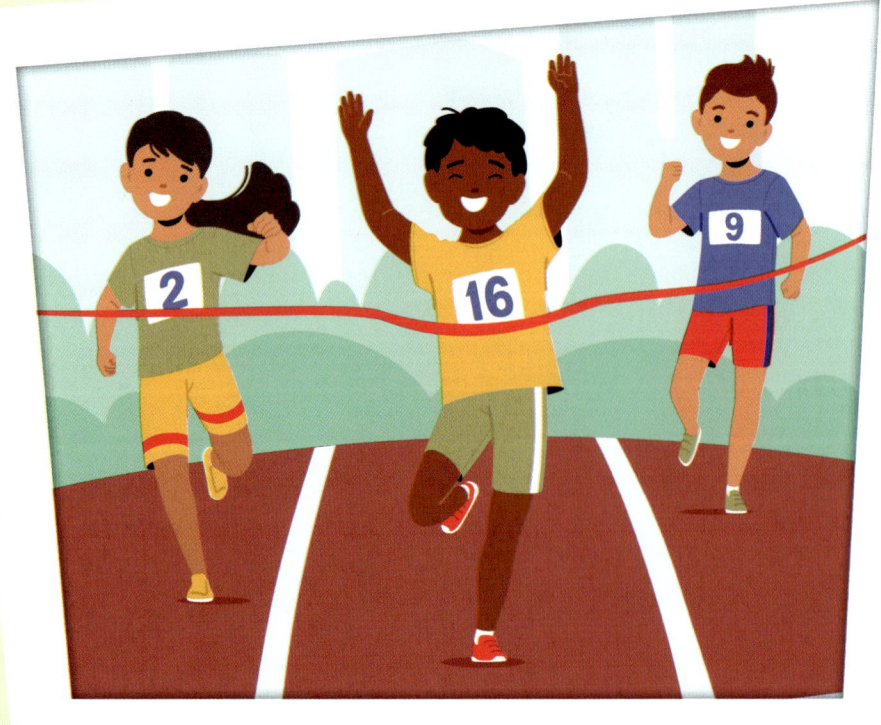

Some people can run really fast.
Others are better at long distances.

Mix and Match

Each sport needs different skills. Here are some skills you can try.

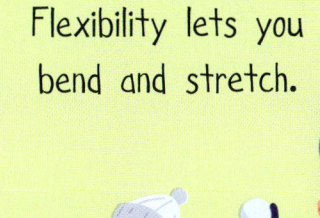

Balance helps you hold your body steady.

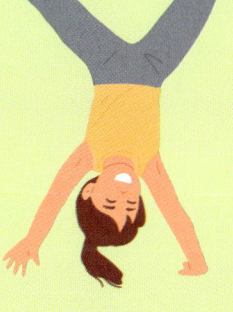

Flexibility lets you bend and stretch.

Coordination lets your body parts work together.

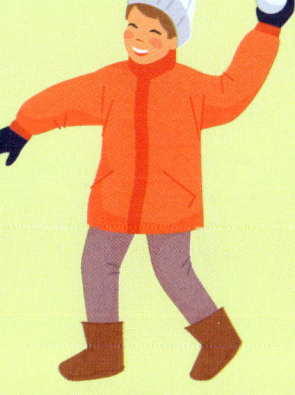

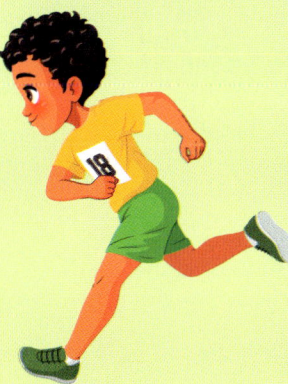

Aim helps you hit a target with a ball or other item.

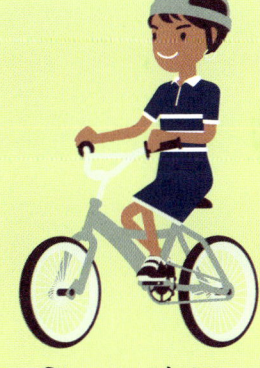

Stamina lets you keep moving without getting tired.

Speed moves you along quickly.

Getting Ready

If you're going to work your body hard, you need to be prepared.

Do a warm-up before you start. It gets your body ready for action! Start with a gentle jog to raise your heart rate. Then swing your arms to loosen up the joints. Do the same with your hips and ankles. Last, stretch to loosen your muscles.

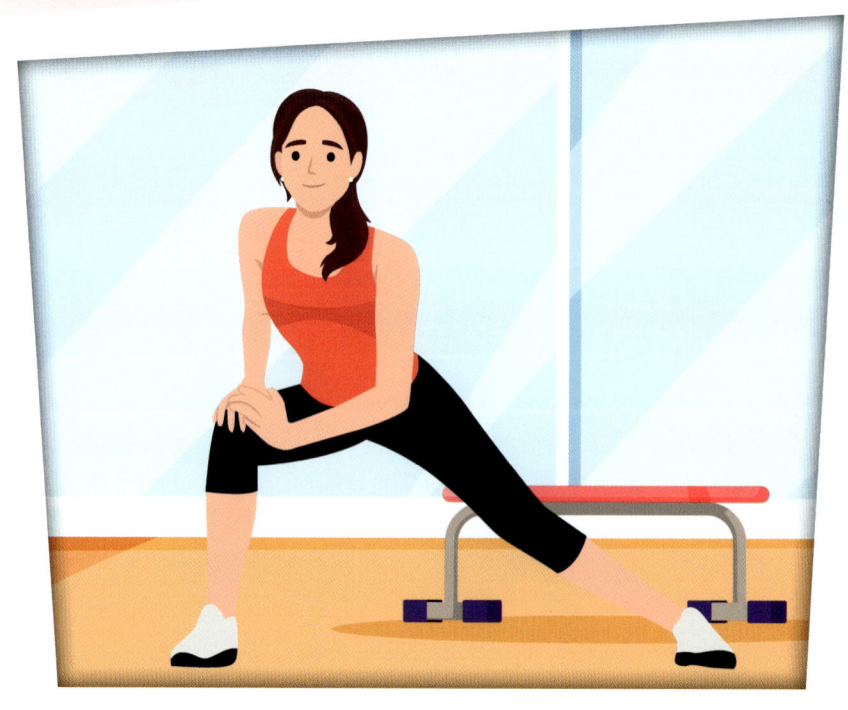

Warming up gets your body ready to work. You're less likely to get injured.

Cooldown

Cooling down is just as important as the warm-up. Jog slowly or walk until you're not panting anymore. Your heart rate will be back to normal now. Then stretch your muscles again. This helps them recover. You'll be ready for the next challenge!

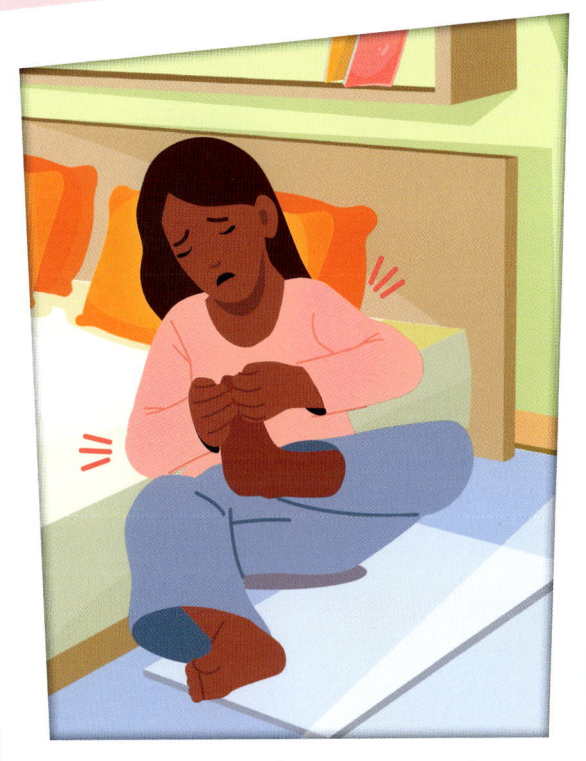

If you don't do a cooldown, your muscles might be sore the next day.

Your warm-up and cooldown should each last for about **5-10** minutes.

Power Up!

**A rocket needs fuel to take off.
Your body needs fuel, too!**

Exercising uses up energy. This energy comes from the food you eat. You need to eat more to replace it. If you choose healthy food, your body will work better! Foods like pasta and oatmeal provide energy. Milk, chicken, and nuts help build muscles.

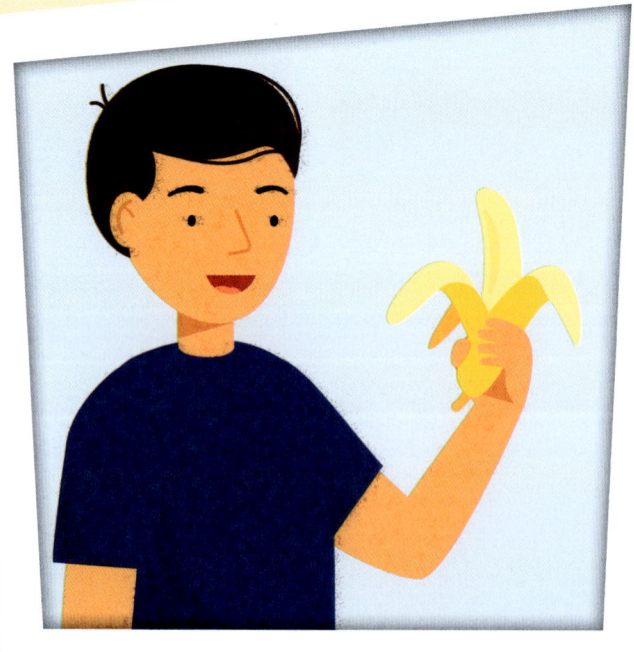

A quick snack will give you a burst
of extra energy. Fruit is a great choice!

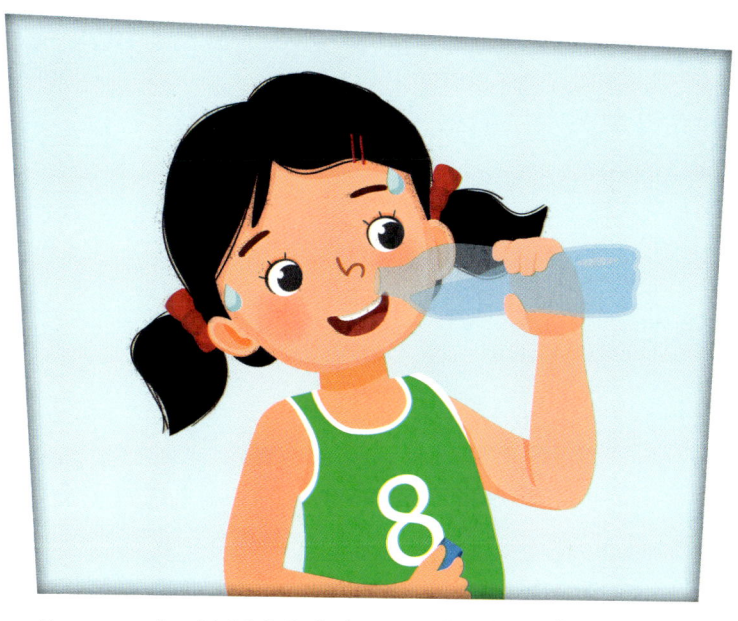

Everyone should drink 6–8 glasses of water a day.
You might need more when you're active.

Drink Water

Athletes often use sports drinks. These have sugar for energy. But most children don't need them. Water is best.

Don't Forget...

When you sweat, your body loses water. You need to replace it by drinking more! Keep a water bottle handy when you're being active. Have a sip whenever you take a break. Have a nice long drink when you're finished.

Active Together

You've decided to become more active. That's great! But what comes next?

Think about ways to work activity into your day. Can you walk or bike instead of driving. Use stairs instead of elevators when you can. Hit the park instead of playing video games. Little bits of exercise can really add up!

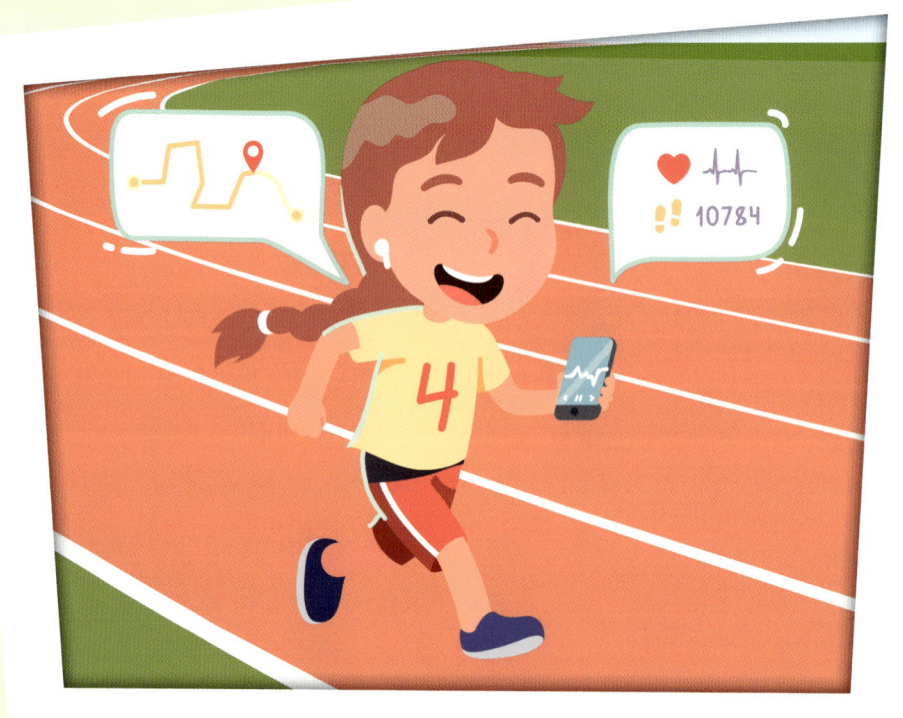

Fitness trackers show you how much activity you've done.

Working Together

It's always easier to do something new when you have company.

Talk to your family about getting active together. You can have fun and keep fit at the same time. You could take a walk. You could go for a family swim. Why not try a new sport together?

Which of these sports uses a ball?

A. ice skating

B. karate

C. tennis

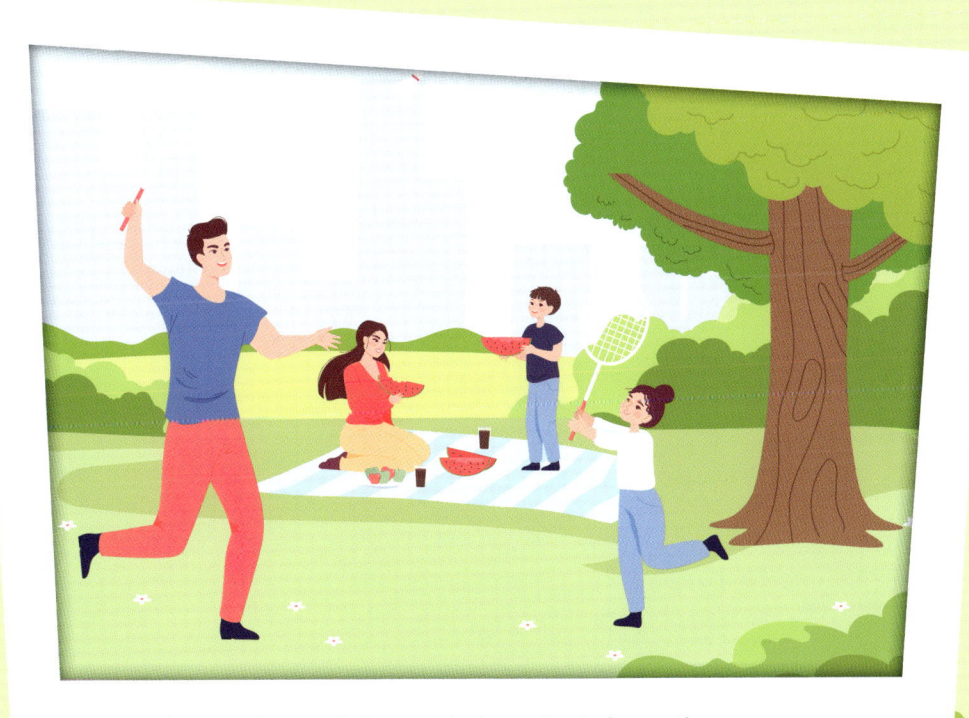

You don't have to be good at sport to have fun being active.

Your Turn!

**You can take charge of staying active!
Here are some ideas.**

1. Keep an activity diary for a few weeks. Write down the active things you do and how long you spend doing them. Then add it all up. Overall, are you active for an hour a day?

2. Help your grown-up make an activity plan for the week. Include the whole family! Think of different ways that you can be active together each day. Include some indoor activities, in case it rains.

Find Out More

Books

Olson, Elsie. Be Well!: *A Hero's Guide to a Healthy Mind and Body (Be Your Best You!)*. Minneapolis, Minn.: Super Sandcastle, 2020.

Susienka, Kristen. *Staying Active and Exercising (Healthy Choices)*. New York: Cavendish Square Publishing, 2021.

Woolley, Katie. *Exercise and Play (My Healthy Life)*. New York: Rosen Publishing, 2024.

Websites

www.bbc.co.uk/bitesize/articles/zbvrcmn#zrc8dp3

kidshealth.org/en/kids/no-sports.html

wonderopolis.org/wonder/why-do-athletes-stretch-before-they-work-out

Glossary

bones the hard, strong body parts that make up the skeleton and hold the body up

cooldown gentle stretches and exercises that help your body wind down after exercise

coordination the way different muscles work together to carry out a complicated movement

energy the power or ability to work or be active; we use energy when we move and grow

flexibility the ability to use the movement of your joints to bend and stretch

heart the organ that pumps blood around the body

joint a place in the body where two parts are connected, such as the elbow or knee

lungs the organs in the chest that take oxygen from the air we breathe in and pass it on to the blood

muscle tissue in the body that squeezes to pull on bones and relaxes to release them

oxygen a gas in the air that humans and animals need to breathe in order to survive

stamina the ability to keep up activity levels for a long time, such as when running a long race

sweat a liquid produced by the skin to cool the body and get rid of waste substances

warm-up getting ready for exercise by raising the heart rate and loosening joints and muscles

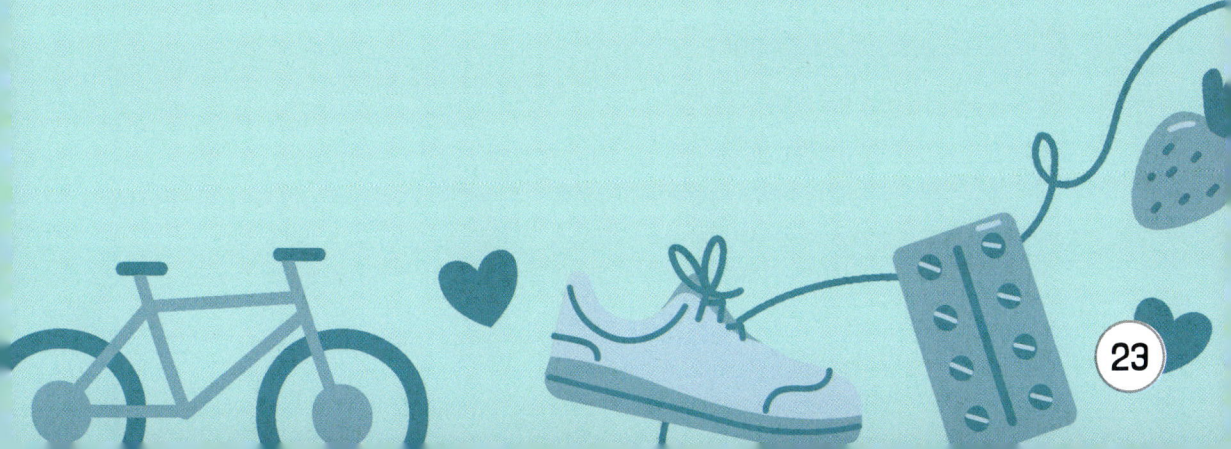

Index

B
biking 5, 6, 12, 20
blood 7, 9
body 4, 5, 6, 7, 8, 9, 10, 12, 14, 15, 16, 18, 19
bones 8, 10, 13
brain 9
breathing 7, 13

C
cooling down 17

D
dancing 4, 5, 11, 12

E
energy 18

F
flexibility 13, 15
food 18

G
getting stronger 7, 8, 10

H
having fun 5, 13, 21
heart 7, 9, 10, 13, 16, 17

J
joints 16
jumping 4, 14

L
lungs 7, 9, 13

M
muscles 7, 8, 9, 10, 13, 16, 17, 18

O
oxygen 7

P
panting 10, 17
playing 11, 12, 13, 20

R
running and jogging 4, 5, 12, 14, 16, 17

S
skills 14, 15
sports 5, 15, 21
stretching 16, 17
sweating 10, 19
swimming 12, 21

W
walking 5, 10, 11, 12, 17, 20, 21
warming up 16, 17
water 19

Answers to questions

page 9: E (exercise boosts your brain and helps keep the heart, lungs, and muscles strong)

page 21: C (tennis balls are small and usually yellow; you need skates for ice skating but no special equipment for karate)